Vegetarian Cookbook Made Easy

Lots of delicious beginner recipes for cooking succulent plant-based dishes. Follow a healthy diet by eating tasty vegetable meals prepared quickly and easily.

Tasty Veggie

1

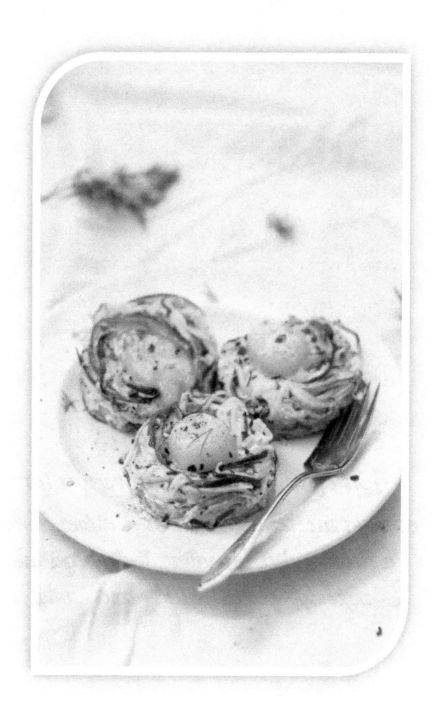

Disclaimer Notice:

Please note the information contained within this document is for educational and entertainment purposes only. All effort has been executed to present accurate, up to date, and reliable, complete information. No warranties of any kind are declared or implied. Readers acknowledge that the author is not engaging in the rendering of legal, financial, medical or professional advice. The content within this book has been derived from various sources. Please consult a licensed professional before attempting any techniques outlined in this book. By reading this document, the reader agrees that under no circumstances is the author responsible for any losses, direct or indirect, which are incurred as a result of the use of information contained within this inaccuracies.

TABLE OF CONTENTS

INTRODUCTION

Vegetarian diets are becoming increasingly popular in the western industrialized nations. Around four percent of the German population also have a meatless diet.

Vegetarianism goes back to the Greek philosopher Pythagoras from the sixth century BC. He wrote the quote: "Everything that humans do to animals comes back to humans." The term vegetarianism comes from the Latin "vegetare" and means "to live" or "to grow".

The numerous scandals surrounding animal products and feed contamination confirm many vegetarians in their decision to eat a meatless diet. Today, many people choose a meat-free or low-meat diet less for philosophical or religious reasons than for concerns about health and the environment. Most vegetarians are also ecologically conscious and prefer organically grown foods.

Forms of vegetarianism

You can live a vegetarian life in different ways. The three most important are:

VEGAN: Vegans only eat plant-based food. They reject any animal-derived substances or products in their food, even honey.

LACTO-VEGETABLE: plant-based food supplemented with milk and dairy products

OVO-LACTO-VEGETABLE: vegetable food with milk, dairy products and eggs

There are also other names. The "pudding vegetarians", for example, do not eat meat, but do not eat health-consciously - with them white flour products, sweets and industrially produced foods are part of their daily menu. In addition to eggs and milk, pisco vegetarians also eat fish. Raw food enthusiasts mainly eat vegetable food in raw form. You don't have to be a vegetarian, though.

BENEFITS OF THE VEGETARIAN DIET

Vegetarians take in a maximum of 30 percent of the food energy they consume daily from fats. For a person who eats a lot of meat on average, this proportion is around 50 percent. The low-fat vegetarian diet is therefore often used as a therapy, for example in the case of lifestyle diseases such as obesity or arteriosclerosis, in which diet plays an important role.

The low proportion of cholesterol in vegetable fats also lowers the risk of arteriosclerosis and cardiovascular diseases. Obesity and heart disease are rare among vegetarians. Most vegetarians, however, are generally very health-conscious - they exercise a lot, smoke little and hardly drink any alcohol.

The carbohydrates contained in cereal products, fruits and vegetables serve vegetarians as the main source of energy. They provide 60 percent of the daily intake. The German Nutrition Society (DGE) recommends that non-vegetarians also consume fat and carbohydrates in a ratio similar to that of the plant-based dieters

.

DISADVANTAGE

A vegetarian diet can lead to an undersupply of vitamin B12. Because this vitamin is almost exclusively contained in animal products.

Meeting iron needs can be problematic without meat as the main supplier, since iron from plant-based foods is less well absorbed by humans than from meat products. Vegetarian women of childbearing age should pay particular attention to an adequate supply of iron.

Iodine, calcium, zinc, vitamin D, riboflavin and certain fatty acids may also be ingested in insufficient amounts.

For vegan there is an even higher risk of developing one or more nutrient deficiencies. A purely vegan diet for the mother during pregnancy can lead to blood formation disorders and severe growth disorders in the child and, among other things, trigger mental retardation. Therefore, as a precaution, the German Nutrition Society advises against a purely vegan diet - especially pregnant women, breastfeeding women and children.

If you want to eat vegan, you should deal intensively with your diet and put your food together consciously. If necessary, it can also be useful to ask your doctor about food supplements (especially vitamin B12, iron, iodine and others) and to have your nutritional requirements checked regularly.

VEGETERIAN BREAKFAST RECIPES

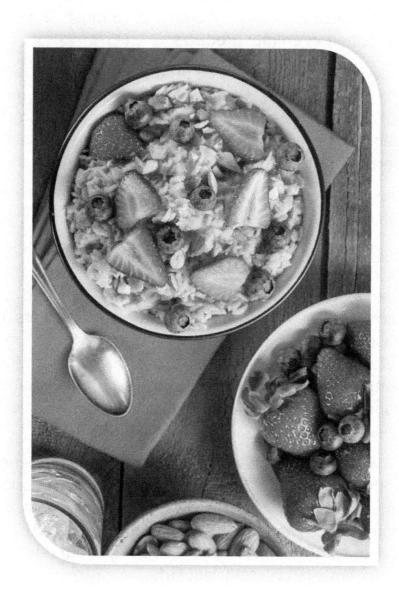

ZUCCHINI JAM

> **Servings:4**

INGREDIENTS

- ✓ 500 g Sour apple
- ✓ 500 g Preserving sugar (2: 1)
- ✓ 50 ml Cater
- ✓ 500 g Zucchini

PREPARATION

- ❖ Wash the zucchini, peel and halve lengthways, remove the seeds and coarsely grate the pulp.

- ❖ Peel and dice the apples. Cover the apples and zucchini with the water in a saucepan and bring to the boil for 8 to 10 minutes over low heat. Add the preserving sugar and cook for another 5 to 10 minutes.

- ❖ Take the jam off the stove. Immediately fill into clean jars and close airtight.

ELDERFLOWER YOGURT

➢ **Servings:4**

INGREDIENTS

✓ 500 ml Milk
✓ 1 cups Natural yoghurt
✓ 4 Pc Elderflower

PREPARATION

❖ Put the milk with the clean elderflower (not washed, just shake dry) in a saucepan and let it boil once, pull it to the side and let it cool down to around 40 ° C. Take the yoghurt out of the refrigerator in good time so that it is at room temperature.

❖ Remove the flowers, possibly pour the milk through a fine sieve and mix well with the yoghurt.

❖ Let the milk-yoghurt mixture (preferably in a mixing bowl) stand in a warm place (at approx. 40-50 ° C) overnight until it has set.

❖ Then store the finished yogurt in the refrigerator for 2-3 days as usual.

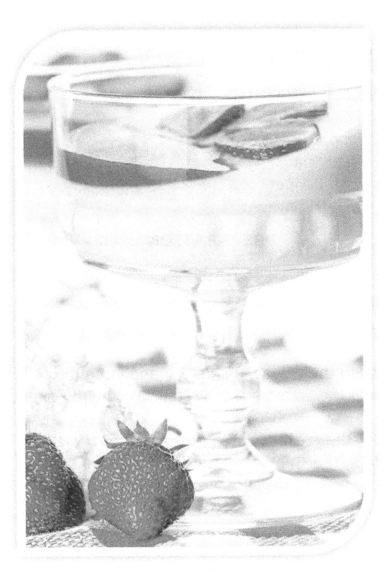

SPRING SPREAD

> **Servings:4**

INGREDIENTS

- ✓ 100 g Potting
- ✓ 6 Pc Cadish
- ✓ 0.5 Federation chives
- ✓ 0.5 Cups cress
- ✓ 2 Tbsp Milk
- ✓ 1 Prize Salt
- ✓ 1 Prize Pepper

PREPARATION

❖ Mix the curd cheese with the milk. Wash the radishes and cut into small cubes.

❖ Wash the chives, shake dry and cut into rolls with the scissors (put 8 stalks of chives aside).

❖ Cut the cress, wash and shake dry, mix the pots, radish pieces, chives and cress together and season to taste with salt and pepper.

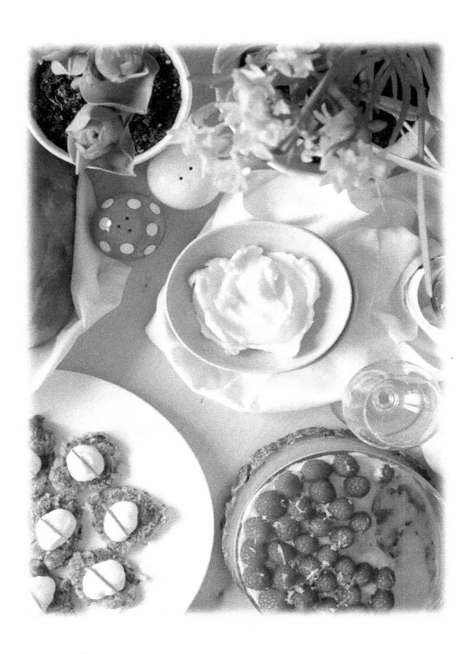

VEGAN CHIA PUDDING

> **Servings:2**

INGREDIENTS

- ✓ 4 Tbsp Chia seeds
- ✓ 250 ml Soy milk
- ✓ 2 TL Agave syrup
- ✓ 1 Prize Cinnamon
- ✓ 1 Prize Cocoa powder
- ✓ Ingredients for serving
- ✓ 2 Tbsp Red currant (or seasonal fruit)
- ✓ 4 Tbsp Cornflakes (vegan)

PREPARATION

❖ Put the soy milk in a small bowl and sweeten to taste, for example with agave syrup.

❖ Mix the chia seeds into the milk while stirring, leave to stand for 10 minutes so that the seeds can unfold nicely. Stir every now and then so that there are no lumps.

❖ You can now season this mixture to taste with cocoa and cinnamon.

❖ Let the pudding stand for at least half an hour so that the seeds can swell properly.

❖ The pudding is served in a glass, the pudding is first poured in. If you wish, you can now top with cornflakes, as well as currants or the favorite fruit you have. Finally, add chia pudding again and serve.

NERVE MUESLI

> ➤ **Servings:1**

INGREDIENTS

- ✓ 1 Pc Baby banana
- ✓ 100 g Wild strawberries
- ✓ 1 Tbsp Sunflower seeds
- ✓ 0.125 l Whole Milk
- ✓ 1 Tbsp Yeast flakes
- ✓ 1 Tbsp Dried wheat germ
- ✓ 1 Tbsp Wheat flakes

PREPARATION

❖ Soak 1 tbsp sunflower seeds for 12 hours. Then let it sprout for 2 days, rinsing twice a day. The germ should be about as long as the core.

❖ Peel the baby banana and cut into a mixing bowl. Clean and add 100 g wild strawberries.

❖ Puree the fruits with the hand blender, pour in 1/8 l milk. Puree 1 tbsp yeast flakes and 1 tbsp wheat germ.

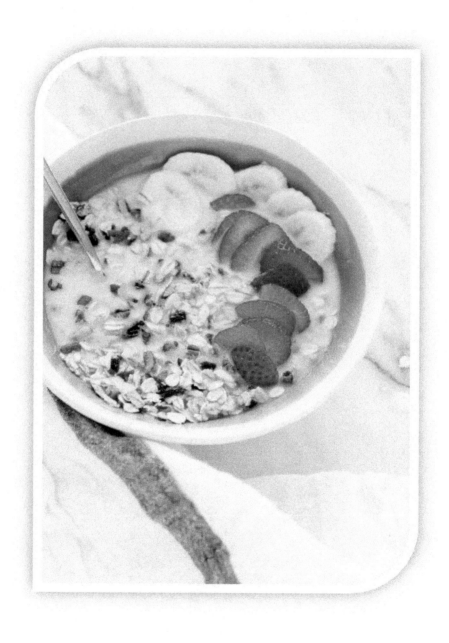

CRUNCHY MUESLI MELBA

> **Servings:1**

INGREDIENTS

- ✓ 2 Tbsp Amaranth cereal
- ✓ 100 G Raspberries
- ✓ 1 TL Honey
- ✓ 1 Pc Blueberries
- ✓ 1 Pc Lemon balm
- ✓ 1 Shot Milk
- ✓ Calculate servings ingredients on the shopping list

PREPARATION

- ❖ Mix all ingredients, arrange in a plate or bowl and garnish with lemon balm if you like.

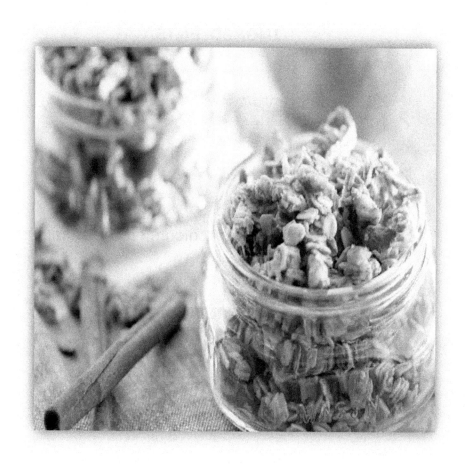

GOOSEBERRY JAM

> **Servings:2**

INGREDIENTS

- ✓ 500 g Gooseberries
- ✓ 1 Pc Vanilla pod
- ✓ 1 Pc Orange
- ✓ 500 g Preserving sugar 1: 1

PREPARATION

- ❖ Wash the gooseberries thoroughly, remove the stalk and flower roots. Squeeze the orange, cut the vanilla pod lengthways and scrape out the pulp.

- ❖ Puree 400 grams of the gooseberries, roughly cut 100 grams of the gooseberries. Put the gooseberry puree, gooseberry pieces, vanilla pulp and the squeezed orange juice in a saucepan. Stir the jam sugar into the mixture and let it boil for 4-6 minutes, take the first jelly sample after 4 minutes (put some of the jam on a cold plate - if the jam stays firm as soon as it has cooled, the jam is ready).

❖ Pour the finished jam into jars rinsed with cold water and close tightly.

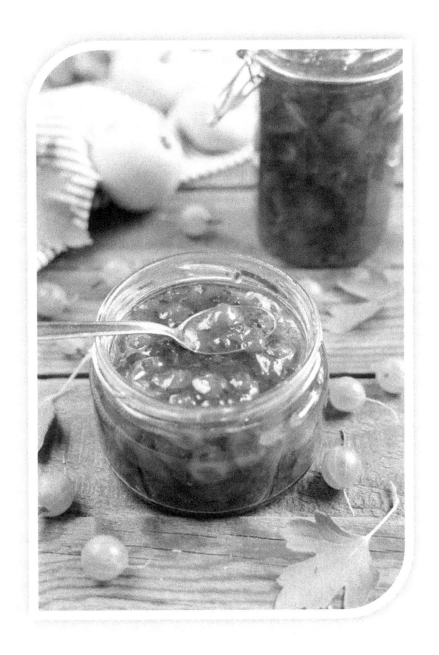

WARM CEREAL

➢ **Servings:4**

INGREDIENTS

✓ 250 g Cereal flakes
✓ 750 ml Skimmed milk
✓ 3 tl Honey
✓ 3 tbsp Raisins
✓ 4 Pc Prunes
✓ 50 g Walnuts, chopped

PREPARATION

❖ Mix the cereal flakes with the skimmed milk, sweeten with honey and place in the unperforated cooking container of the steamer.

❖ Finely chop the raisins and prunes and mix into the flakes. Let the mixture steam for 15 minutes.

❖ Chop the walnuts into fine pieces and mix with the rest of the ingredients.

VEGETERIAN LUNCH RECIPES

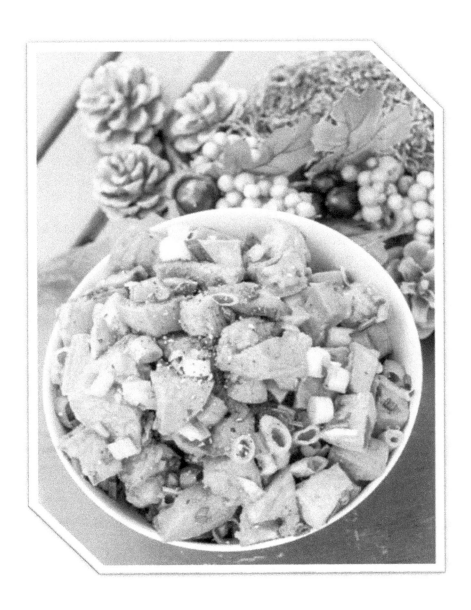

ORIENTAL COUSCOUS PAN WITH VEGETABLES

> **Servings:4**

INGREDIENTS

- ✓ 200 g Melanzani
- ✓ 200 g White cabbage
- ✓ 150 g Tomatoes
- ✓ 250 g Carrots
- ✓ 2 Pc Onions
- ✓ 2 Pc Garlic cloves
- ✓ 250 ml Clear vegetable soup
- ✓ 300 g Couscous
- ✓ 5 Tbsp Olive oil
- ✓ 150 g Canned Chickpeas
- ✓ 200 ml Carrot Juice
- ✓ 1 Prize Salt
- ✓ 2 TL Harissa (from the tube)
- ✓ 25 g Pine Nuts
- ✓ 4 Stg Mint
- ✓ 1 Prize Pepper
- ✓ 1 Shot Lemon Juice

PREPARATION

❖ For this oriental dish, first wash the aubergines, carrots and tomatoes thoroughly, drain them and set them aside. Drain the chickpeas through a sieve, rinse with water and drain.

❖ Now cut the tomatoes and aubergines into bite-sized pieces and the carrots into thin slices. Then remove the leaves from the cabbage and cut out the thick ribs - cut the rest into fine strips.

❖ Now peel and finely chop the onions and garlic. Heat the clear vegetable soup in a saucepan, switch off the stove again and add the couscous, cover and leave to swell for 5-10 minutes - until all the liquid is absorbed.

❖ Heat 3 tablespoons of oil in a large pan (for example a wok) and fry the cut vegetables with the garlic and onions for 4-5 minutes. Empty the chickpeas along with the carrot juice and pine nuts over the vegetables. Season the whole thing with salt and harissa (hot spice paste) and let it stew for 10 minutes over a low flame.

❖ In the meantime, wash the mint, shake it dry and cut the plucked leaves into fine strips -

these are added to the couscous together with 2 tablespoons of oil.

❖ Mix the finished couscous with the fried vegetables, season again with salt, pepper and a dash of lemon juice (or lime juice) if necessary and serve on 4 plates.

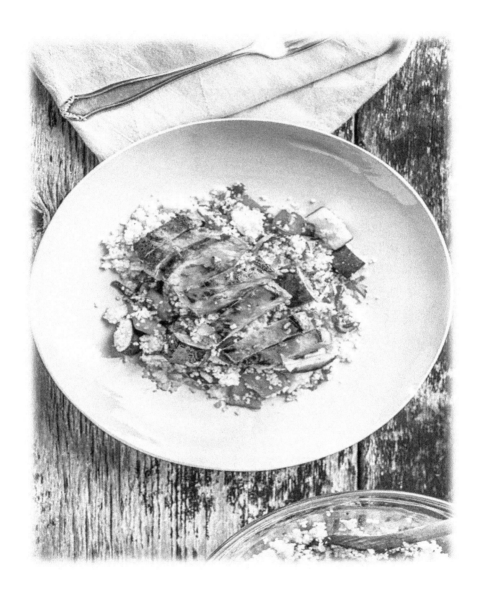

ERDÄPFELLAIBCHEN

> **Servings:4**

INGREDIENTS

- ✓ 8 Pc Potatoes (medium)
- ✓ 200 g Potting
- ✓ 1 Prize Nutmeg, ground
- ✓ 1 Prize Salt
- ✓ 1 Prize Pepper
- ✓ 1 Pc Onion
- ✓ 1 Pc Egg
- ✓ 2 Tbsp Parsley, Chopped
- ✓ 4 Tbs Poil

PREPARATION

❖ Wash the potatoes, cut the larger ones in half lengthways and cook in boiling water for about 30 minutes until they are soft. Peel off the skin and mash with the potato masher (or use a fork).

❖ Peel the onion and cut into small cubes. Heat the oil and steam the onion pieces in it until translucent, then add to the potatoes. Add the saucepan, egg and parsley and season everything with salt, pepper and nutmeg, then knead into an even dough.

❖ Shape patties of the same size with wet hands. Heat the oil in a non-stick pan and fry the potato patties for 5 minutes on each side.

ZUCCHINI POTATO PANCAKES

> **Servings:2**

INGREDIENTS

- ✓ 350 g Potatoes
- ✓ 450 g Zucchini
- ✓ 3 Tbsp Oatmeal
- ✓ 1 Pc Onion
- ✓ 1 Tbsp Sunflower oil
- ✓ 1 Prize Salt
- ✓ 1 Prize Nutmeg, Ground
- ✓ 1 Prize Paprika Powder
- ✓ 2 Pc Eggs
- ✓ 2 Tbsp Flour
- ✓ 1 prize Pepper White

PREPARATION

❖ Peel the potatoes and grate them finely. Wash the zucchini and grate as well. Mix both, salt and let steep for 10 minutes.

❖ Peel the onion and use the chopper to make it almost a pulp.

❖ Tip the potato and zucchini mixture into a sieve, strain and squeeze out. Put in a bowl and mix with the onions, oat flakes, eggs and flour, season with salt, pepper, paprika and nutmeg.

❖ Heat a little oil in a non-stick pan. With the help of 2 tablespoons, add the potato-zucchini mixture to the pan, press flat and fry until golden brown on both sides. Put on kitchen paper and degrease.

BAKED AUBERGINES

➢ **Servings:4**

INGREDIENTS

✓ 2 Pc Melanzani
✓ 3 Pc Eggs
✓ 1 Cup Flour
✓ 1 Cup Breadcrumbs
✓ 1 Prize Salt
✓ 300 g Rapeseed oil

PREPARATION

❖ Wash and dry aubergines. Cut off both ends, cut the rest into slices of about 1 cm.

❖ Beat the eggs in a bowl and whisk with the salt. Put the flour and breadcrumbs each on a plate.

❖ First turn the eggplant slices in the flour, then pull them through the egg mixture and finally press them into the breadcrumbs from both sides.

❖ Let the oil heat up in a high pan (or heat the fat in the deep fryer) and fry the aubergines in it on both sides (2 minutes each).

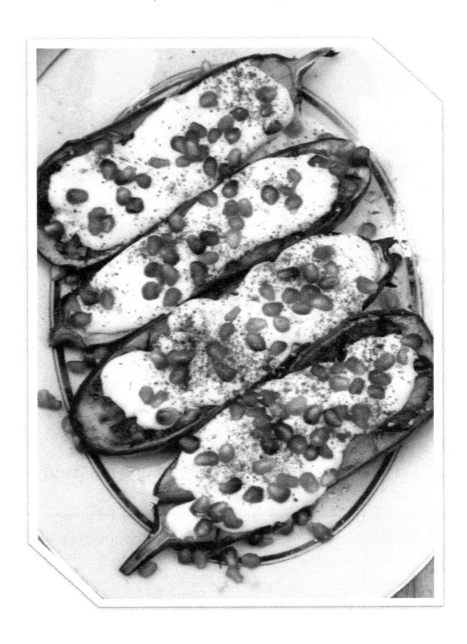

ITALIAN GNOCCHI

➢ **Servings:4**

INGREDIENTS

✓ 1 kg Gnocchi
✓ Ingredients sauce
✓ 2 Pc Zucchini
✓ 1 Pc Melanzani
✓ 2 Pc Garlic cloves
✓ 1 Pc Spring onion
✓ 30 g Thyme
✓ 100 g Tomatoes, dried
✓ 1 Prize Salt
✓ 1 Prize Pepper

PREPARATION

❖ Bring water (with a pinch of salt) to a boil. As soon as the water boils you can add the gnocchi and wait for them to rise to the surface. Attention! The gnocchi will be ready after about a minute. Then strain, rinse with cool water and drain.

❖ Now it goes on with the sauce: Cut the aubergine and zucchini into pieces about 2cm in size. Then peel the garlic and cut into thin slices. The spring onions should also be cleaned and then cut into coarse slices. Then the tomatoes have to be cut into 1cm wide pieces. Finally, the thyme leaves are plucked and roughly chopped.

❖ Now continue in the pan: fry the aubergines and zucchini in 3 tablespoons of oil over high heat until golden brown and season with salt and pepper as desired. Then add the spring onion and garlic. Stir in thyme, gnocchi and tomatoes and refine everything with salt and pepper.

ASIAN RICE PAN

> **Servings:4**

INGREDIENTS

- ✓ 200 g Basmati rice
- ✓ 50 g Cashew nuts
- ✓ 50 g Carrots
- ✓ 50 g Zucchini
- ✓ 50 g Bean sprouts
- ✓ 30 g Morels
- ✓ 1 Pc Ginger, small
- ✓ 3 Tbsp Soy sauce
- ✓ 1 Tbsp Curry paste
- ✓ 2 Msp Chilli powder
- ✓ 1 Tbsp Lemon juice
- ✓ 3 Tbsp Frying oil

PREPARATION

❖ Prepare rice: measure the water according to the instructions on the packet and bring to the boil. Add the basmati rice, turn off the heat and let the rice soak for about 20 minutes (or according to the package instructions).

❖ In the meantime, peel the carrots and wash them into thin strips or zucchini and cut into small pieces. Peel the ginger and grate it with a grater.

❖ Heat 2 tablespoons of oil in a coated pan and fry the carrots in it. Then add the zucchini, bean sprouts, morels and cashew nuts and continue frying.

❖ Add the finished rice and fry with another tablespoon of oil.

❖ Deglaze with soy sauce, then add ginger, curry paste, chili powder and lemon juice; serve immediately.

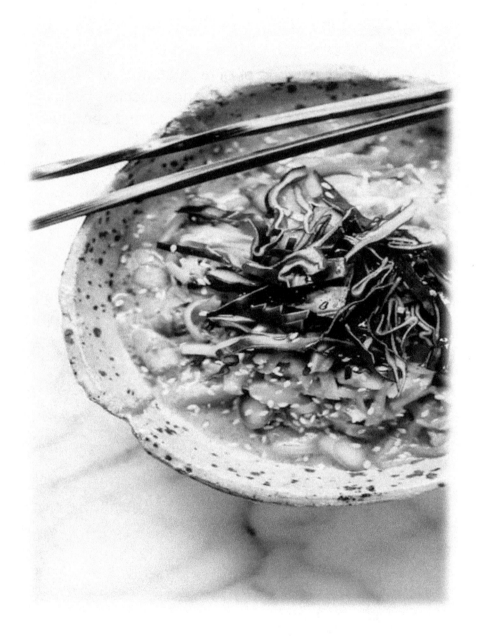

SPICY PANCAKES

> **Servings:4**

INGREDIENTS

- ✓ 3 Pc Onion
- ✓ 400 g Mushrooms
- ✓ 4 Tbsp Sour cream
- ✓ 1 Prize Cayenne pepper
- ✓ 1 Prize Salt
- ✓ 1 Prize Paprika powder
- ✓ 3 Pc Peppers, red
- ✓ 2 Tbsp Olive oil
- ✓ 2 Tbsp Soy sauce
- ✓ 150 g Arugula

Ingredients for the dough

- ✓ 25 g Flour
- ✓ 4 Pc Eggs
- ✓ 500 ml Milk
- ✓ 1 Prize Salt
- ✓ 3 Tbsp Clarified butter

PREPARATION

❖ First prepare the pancake batter: sift the flour into a bowl. Add the milk, eggs and salt and mix everything into a liquid, even dough. Heat the fat in a pan and fry 8 thin pancakes one after the other - it is best to pour the dough into the pan with a soup ladle and fry briefly on both sides. Stack the finished pancakes on a plate and keep warm.

❖ Now peel the onions and cut them into cubes. Halve the bell pepper, cut out the core and white partitions, wash and cut into small cubes. Clean the mushrooms and cut them in slices. Wash the rocket and shake dry.

❖ Then heat the olive oil in a pan and fry the onion and pepper cubes in it, then briefly sauté the mushroom slices. Season with paprika powder, cayenne pepper and salt.

❖ Spread 3 tablespoons of fried vegetables on each pancake and drizzle with a little soy sauce. Then spread the washed rocket on top and add a tablespoon of sour cream. Roll up the pancakes and fill the remaining pancakes as described.

SLOPPY JOES

> **Servings:4**

INGREDIENTS

- ✓ 6 TL Chili sauce
- ✓ 500 g Tofu, firm
- ✓ 6 TL Ketchup
- ✓ 1 TL Vegetable oil for the pan
- ✓ 0.5 TL Salt
- ✓ 1 Pc Paprika, green
- ✓ 1 Pc Medium onion
- ✓ 1 prize Pepper
- ✓ 4 Pc Burger bun

PREPARATION

- ❖ To do this, peel and finely chop the onions, wash the green peppers, remove the stalk, core and cut just as finely.

- ❖ Now heat the oil in a large frying pan over medium heat and fry the finely chopped onion and pepper pieces for about 5 minutes - stirring occasionally.

- ❖ Chop the tofu and add it to the pan - fry for another 15 minutes, until the tofu is almost overcooked.
- ❖ Now add the ketchup (or a homemade tomato sauce), chilli sauce, salt and pepper and cook over low heat until the mixture is thoroughly heated. If necessary, add a little water if the mixture is still too dry.

- ❖ Lightly fry the burger buns cut in half on the cut side (preferably directly in the pan or on a toaster) and spread the tofu sauce on top with a spoon.

VEGETERIAN DINNER RECIPES

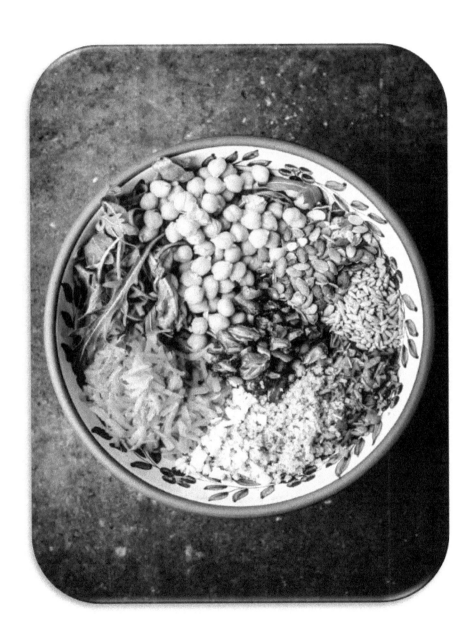

VEGETARIAN MEAT STRIPS FROM ZURICH

> **Servings:4**

INGREDIENTS

- ✓ 1 TL Butter
- ✓ 150 ml Well Seasoned Vegetable Bouillon
- ✓ 1 Tbsp Flour
- ✓ 1 Federation Peterli Smooth-Leaved
- ✓ 600 g Mixed Mushrooms (mushrooms, shiitake, oyster mushrooms
- ✓ 200 ml Sauce Cream
- ✓ 4 Pc Shallots
- ✓ 150 ml White Wine

PREPARATION

❖ Peel and finely chop shallots. Clean the mushrooms well (do not wash) and cut into slices.

❖ Melt the butter in a frying pan. Add shallots and sauté until translucent. Dust the mushrooms with flour and mix everything well. Add mushrooms to the pan and fry well over high heat, stirring constantly.

- ❖ Reduce heat. Deglaze with wine and bouillon. Reduce to half over medium heat.
- ❖ Add the cream for the sauce. Mix well. Simmer over low heat until a creamy sauce is formed. Arrange on plates and sprinkle with chopped parsley.

ZUCCHINI-SPAGHETTI

➢ **Servings:2**

INGREDIENTS

✓ 500 g Cherry tomatoes
✓ 1 Pc Chilli Pepper, Red
✓ 2 Pc Garlic Cloves
✓ 2 Tbsp Olive Oil
✓ 80 g Parmesan, Grated
✓ 2 Tbsp Pesto, Red
✓ 1 Prize Pepper
✓ 70 g Pine Nuts
✓ 1 Prize Salt
✓ 3 Pc Zucchini

PREPARATION

❖ For the zucchini spaghetti, wash the zucchini thoroughly and cut into strips.

❖ Then peel and finely chop the fresh garlic cloves for the sauce. Wash the chilli, cut lengthways, core and finely chop.

- ❖ Now lightly fry the garlic cubes with the chilli and pine nuts in a pan with a little olive oil for about 5 minutes.

- ❖ Meanwhile, wash the cherry tomatoes and cut them in half. Rinse the basil leaves, shake dry and finely chop. Stir both together with the pesto into the sauce and let it simmer for about 5 minutes.

- ❖ Then stir in the zucchini strips and simmer for another 15 minutes on low heat.

- ❖ Finally season well with salt and pepper and sprinkle with a little parmesan.

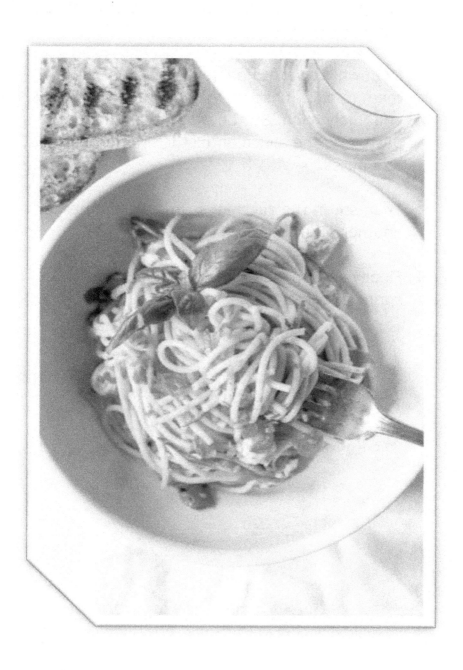

ZUCCHINI SPAGHETTI WITH TOMATO SAUCE

➢ **Servings:1**

INGREDIENTS

- ✓ 1 Tbsp Ajvar
- ✓ 1 Tbsp Basil
- ✓ 8 Pc Cherry Tomatoes
- ✓ 1 Tbsp Cream Cheese
- ✓ 1 Pc Cove of Garlic
- ✓ 1 Tbsp Olive Oil
- ✓ 1 Prize Pepper
- ✓ 1 Prize Salt
- ✓ 1 Pc Zucchini
- ✓ 1 Pc Onion

PREPARATION

❖ For the zucchini spaghetti with tomato sauce, first turn the zucchini into thin spaghetti using a spiral cutter. Peel the fresh onion and cut into fine strips. Then peel and finely chop the clove of garlic.

❖ Now sauté the onion and garlic cubes in a pan with a little olive oil for about 3 minutes until translucent. Stir in the creamy cream cheese and ajvar, simmer for about 3 minutes.

❖ Now stir the zucchini spaghetti into the sauce, sauté for about 5 minutes and season well with salt and pepper.

❖ Then wash the cherry tomatoes, cut in half and stir into the sauce. Season to taste with basil and serve immediately warm.

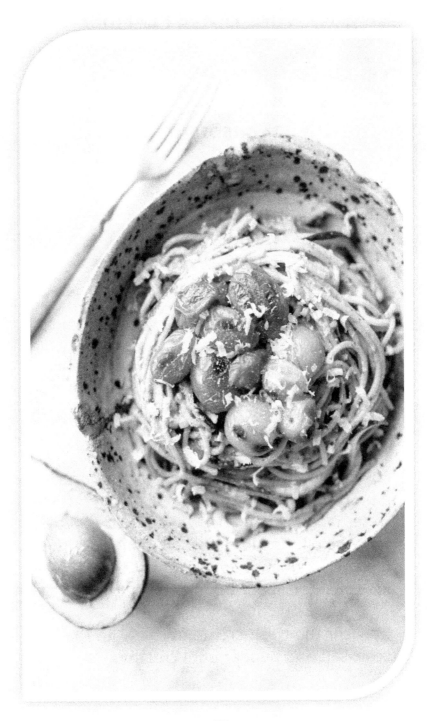

ZUCCHINI TARTE FLAMBÉE

➢ **Servings:2**

INGREDIENTS

✓ 270 g Creme Fraiche Cheese
✓ 20 g Yeast, Fresh
✓ 250 g Flour
✓ 2 Tbsp Olive Oil
✓ 1 Prize Pepper
✓ 0.5 TL Salt
✓ 1 TL Lemon Peel
✓ 2 Pc Zucchini

PREPARATION

❖ For the dough, first mix the flour with the salt in a bowl. Dissolve the fresh yeast with 120 ml of water in a bowl and add to the flour together with the oil. Knead the whole thing with the mixer to a smooth dough. Cover the dough and let it rest for about 30 minutes in a warm place.

❖ Now stir the fresh crème fraiche with the lemon zest, salt and pepper until creamy.

- ❖ Then wash the fresh zucchini and use the peeler to slice lengthways into wide, thin slices.
- ❖ Then divide the dough into 4 pieces and roll out thinly with the rolling pin on a floured work surface. Place the flatbreads on baking sheets lined with baking paper and brush each with the crème fraîche and top with the zucchini strips.

- ❖ Then bake the zucchini tarte flambée in the oven at 250 degrees (convection 230 degrees) for about 15 minutes until crispy.

COURGETTE OMELETTE WITH PUMPKIN SEED OIL

> **Servings:6**

INGREDIENTS

- ✓ 4 Tbsp Butter
- ✓ 9 Pc Eggs
- ✓ 2 Pc Fresh Zucchini
- ✓ 3 Tbsp Herbs, Chopped
- ✓ 1 shot Pumpkin Seed Oil
- ✓ 60 g Parmesan, Freshly Grated
- ✓ 1 Prize Salt Vepper

PREPARATION

❖ Wash and dry the zucchini, cap the ends and cut into thin slices. Whisk the eggs with the parmesan and herbs.

❖ Mix the courgette slices into the egg mixture and season well with salt and pepper.

❖ Let the butter get hot in a large pan and add the egg mixture. Let it bake a little, then put the lid on and let it set over a mild heat (takes about 12-15 minutes).

❖ Let the omelette slide onto a platter, cut open like pieces of cake and drizzle with pumpkin seed oil.

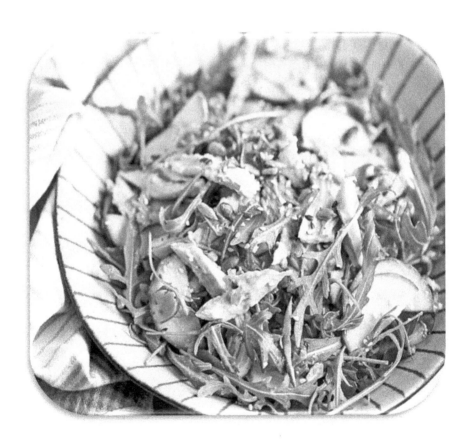

ZUCCHETTI CHEESE SALAD

> **Servings:4**

INGREDIENTS

- ✓ 2 Tbsp Vinegar
- ✓ 1 Tbsp Capers
- ✓ 200 g Cheese (Emmentaler)
- ✓ 4 Tbsp Oil
- ✓ 1 Prize Salt Pepper
- ✓ 1 Federation Chives
- ✓ 1 TL Tustard
- ✓ 0.5 TL Thyme
- ✓ 250 g Zucchini
- ✓ 1 Pc Onion (medium)

PREPARATION

- ❖ Cut the washed courgette into thin strips. Dice the peeled onion.

- ❖ Briefly fry the onions and courgettes in a pan with 1 tablespoon of oil, sprinkle with salt, pepper and thyme and cook covered for 10 minutes.

- ❖ For the marinade, mix 2 tablespoons of oil, vinegar, onion, mustard and finely chopped capers and season with salt and pepper.
- ❖ Cut the cheese into 4 cm long strips, place over the courgette strips, pour the marinade over them and leave to stand for 1 hour, covered.

ZUCCHETTI VEGETABLES WITH ARUGULA

> **Servings:4**

INGREDIENTS

- ✓ 3 Between basil
- ✓ 1 Pc Chili
- ✓ 2 Federation spring onions
- ✓ 3 Pc Garlic cloves
- ✓ 50 ml Olive oil
- ✓ 0.5 TL Pepper
- ✓ 100 g Arugula
- ✓ 0.5 TL Salt
- ✓ 8 Between thyme
- ✓ 500 g Zucchini

PREPARATION

❖ Remove the stalk from the courgette, prepare the spring onions and garlic. Divide the courgettes into fine wheels, roughly chop the onions and garlic. Wash and core the chilli pepper and dice very finely.

❖ Heat the olive oil in a frying pan or wok and fry the spring onions, garlic, chilli and courgettes in it. After about 4 minutes add the thyme, rosemary and salt and pepper and mix all ingredients well. Fry the vegetables for another 5 minutes.

❖ Meanwhile, wash the rocket and drain well. Now add the rocket and basil to the pan and continue frying for a short time. Serve the dish warm as a starter or as a delicious side dish.

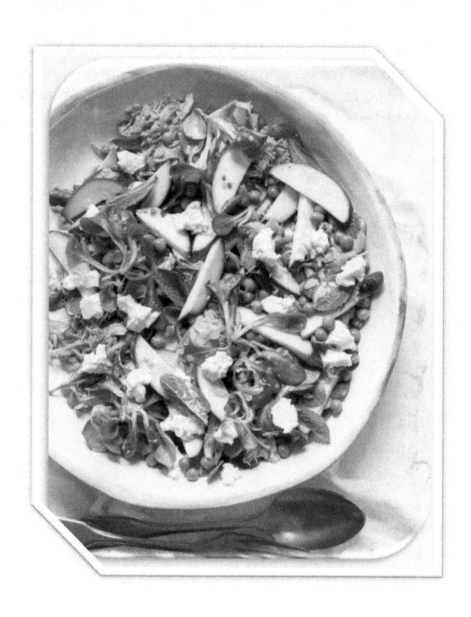

ZAZIKI

> **Servings:5**

INGREDIENTS

- ✓ 1 TL Vinegar
- ✓ 2 Pc Cucumber
- ✓ 500 g Yogurt
- ✓ 4 Pc Garlic cloves
- ✓ 2 TL Olive oil
- ✓ 1 prize Pepper
- ✓ 1 prize Salt
- ✓ 1 prize Sugar

PREPARATION

- ❖ Divide the peeled cucumber in the middle, remove the seeds and grate. Squeeze out the remaining liquid from the cucumber, season with salt and set aside.

- ❖ Then finely chop the peeled garlic. Combine the grated cucumber, yogurt and garlic in a bowl.

❖ Mix the tzaziki with vinegar and olive oil and season with salt, sugar and pepper. Then put in the fridge and let it steep.

VEGETERIAN DESSERT RECIPE

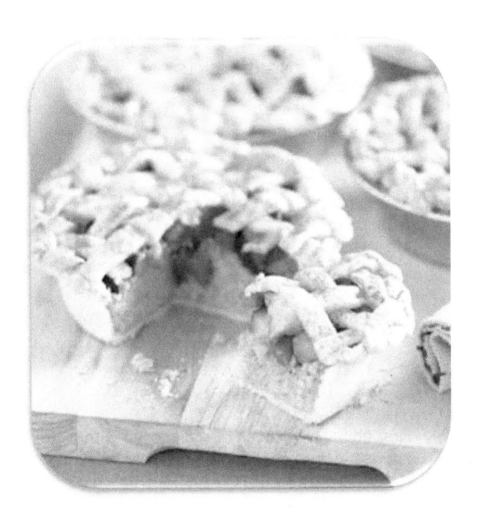

PLUM DUMPLINGS

> **Servings:4**

INGREDIENTS

- ✓ 100 g Butter
- ✓ 60 g Butter, liquid
- ✓ 4 Pc Egg yolk
- ✓ 800 g Potatoes, floury-boiling
- ✓ 6 Tbsp Flour
- ✓ 1 prize Salt
- ✓ 4 Tbsp Wheat semolina
- ✓ 1 prize Sugar
- ✓ 12 Pcp lums

PREPARATION

❖ First boil the potatoes in a saucepan with water until soft, then peel them and squeeze them into a bowl in a press.

❖ Mix the potatoes with the melted butter, egg yolks, flour, salt and semolina. Let the dough rest for a few minutes.

- ❖ Now cut the plums and remove the stones.
- ❖ Shape the dough into balls the size of a plum, press flat and wrap a plum in it. Then turn the dough again into dumplings.

- ❖ Bring salted water to the boil in a saucepan and let the dumplings simmer for about 10 minutes.

- ❖ Meanwhile, melt the 100 g butter in a pan and add the breadcrumbs - add a pinch of sugar to taste.

- ❖ Put the dumplings from the water in the pan and screw in with the crumb mixture.

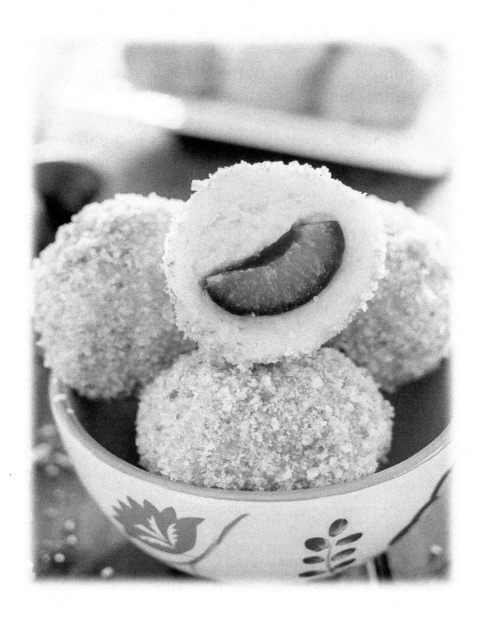

WATERMELON SORBET

> **Servings:4**

INGREDIENTS

✓ 1 Pc Mini watermelon
✓ 1 prize Salt
✓ 800 g Watermelon (weighed without peel)
✓ 2 Pc Lemons

PREPARATION

❖ Loosen the red pulp from the melon, remove the black seeds as much as possible, dice and puree briefly with the hand blender.

❖ Put the resulting mass through a fine sieve (if you have time you can also put a piece of kitchen paper in a sieve, pour in the mass and wait until it is done - then you really only have the pure juice) there should be about 500ml of melon juice left be.

❖ Dissolve 20 grams of powdered sugar (for those who like it refreshing, if you want a sweet sorbet then add 40 grams of powdered sugar) in the melon juice while stirring and add a pinch of salt.

❖ Now squeeze 2 lemons and stir into the melon juice, now season the whole thing - if it still tastes a bit cucumber-like, you can add a little lemon juice.

❖ Pour the liquid into a flat mold and freeze in the refrigerator, stir every 15-20 minutes from the corners to the center with a fork, freeze to the desired firmness and serve or put in a freezer and store in the freezer until use (before Let serve defrost for a few minutes).

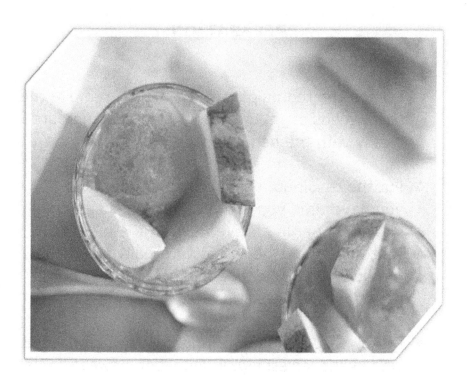

WHOLE GRAIN CREPES WITH FRUITS

➢ **Servings:4**

INGREDIENTS

- 2 Pc Apples
- 2 Pc Eggs
- 120 g Strawberries
- 2 Pc Kiwi
- 70 ml Milk
- 200 ml Mineral water
- 2 Tbsp Oil
- 1 TL Sweetener / or honey
- 200 g Whole wheat flour
- 1 TL Sugar

Ingredients at will

- Bullet Ice cream of your choice (ice cream)
- 1 Tbsp Honey
- 1 Bch Vanilla yogurt

PREPARATION

❖ Wash, peel and core the apples, cut into small pieces and caramelize with sugar.

❖ Carefully mix the flour with the eggs, water, milk and sweetener and stir to form a dough.

❖ Put the oil in the pan and pour in a little batter.

❖ After about a minute, turn the crepes and remove when both sides are golden brown.

❖ Wash, peel and dice the kiwi.

❖ Wash the strawberries and cut them in half.

❖ Mix the fruits.

❖ Put the crepes on a plate, fill with the fruit and close.

TÜRGGERIBEL

> **Servings:4**

INGREDIENTS

- ✓ 100 g Butter
- ✓ 400 g Corn semolina, such as Rheintaler Ribel
- ✓ 200 ml Milk
- ✓ 2 Tbsp Oil
- ✓ 1.5 TL Salt
- ✓ 400 ml Water

PREPARATION

- ❖ Bring semolina, water, milk and salt to the boil in a saucepan and let soak for about 30 minutes.

- ❖ Then place in a pan with heated fat, turn and stir until lumps form.

- ❖ Gradually stir in butter. As soon as the balls have formed (after about 20 minutes), the ribel is ready.

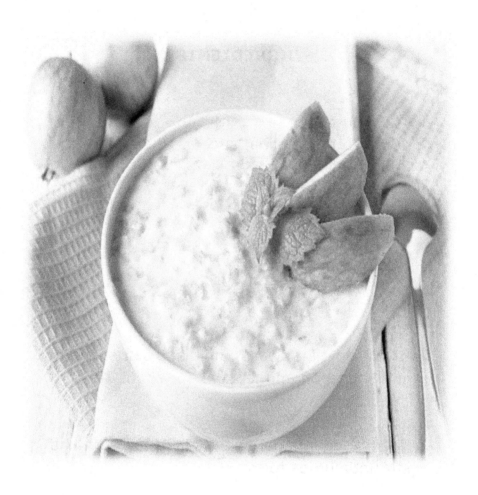

SWEET APPLE COMPOTE

> **Servings:4**

INGREDIENTS

- ✓ 8 Pc Apples
- ✓ 4 Pc Cloves
- ✓ 1 l Water
- ✓ 1 prize Cinnamon
- ✓ 2 Pc Cinnamon sticks
- ✓ 2 Tbsp Lemon juice
- ✓ 1 Pc Lemon peel
- ✓ 120 g Sugar

PREPARATION

- ❖ Let the water with the cloves, cinnamon sticks and a piece of lemon peel boil for 5 minutes. Then pull out the spices with a sieve.

- ❖ Peel the apples, remove the core and cut into approx. 1/2 cm wide wedges. Put the apple wedges together with the sugar in the boiling water and let the apples cook until soft.

❖ Then let cool for a few minutes, add a dash of lemon juice and a pinch of cinnamon and serve.

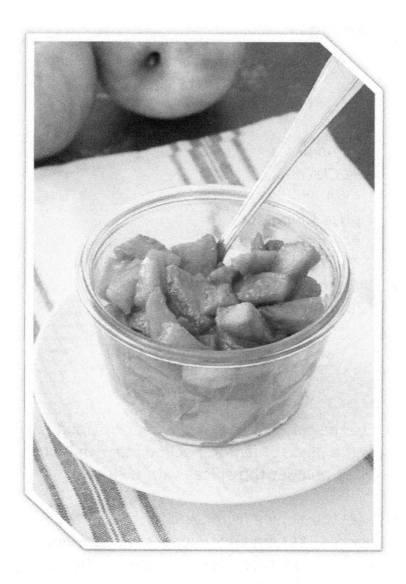

SWEET FLAMBÉED BANANAS

> **Servings:4**

INGREDIENTS

- ✓ 4 Pc Bananas
- ✓ 0.25 Fl Cherry liqueur or a Grand Marnier
- ✓ 4 Tbsp Forest honey

Ingredients tip

- ✓ 1 Cup Fresh raspberries
- ✓ 4 Bullet vanilla ice-cream

PREPARATION

- ❖ The whole bananas are placed on the grill unpeeled. They are grilled until the skin is soft and dark.

- ❖ Now the hot bananas are carefully placed on a plate and halved lengthways.

❖ The banana halves are drizzled or poured with the liqueur on the inside. Then the liqueur is lit on the banana halves. Please keep a safe distance to avoid burns!

❖ As soon as the flame has gone out, you can refine the bananas with a large spoon of liquid forest honey.

❖ Have fun trying it out and en guata!

GRILLED SWEET APRICOTS

> **Servings:6**

INGREDIENTS

- ✓ 18 Pc Apricots
- ✓ 12 Between rosemary
- ✓ Ingredients orange syrup
- ✓ 60 g Butter
- ✓ 4 Tbsp Honey
- ✓ 1 Between mint
- ✓ 1 Pc Orange (juice)
- ✓ 150 ml Peach liquor

PREPARATION

❖ Wash the apricots briefly and then cut in half, stone and skewer 3 halves each onto a sprig of rosemary.

❖ For the orange syrup, reduce the honey and orange juice in a small saucepan over medium heat. Add the butter, mint and peach liqueur, mix and simmer for about 5 minutes until a creamy orange syrup is formed.

❖ Fry the apricot skewers on the grill over high heat for 5 minutes and serve the hot skewers with a little orange syrup.

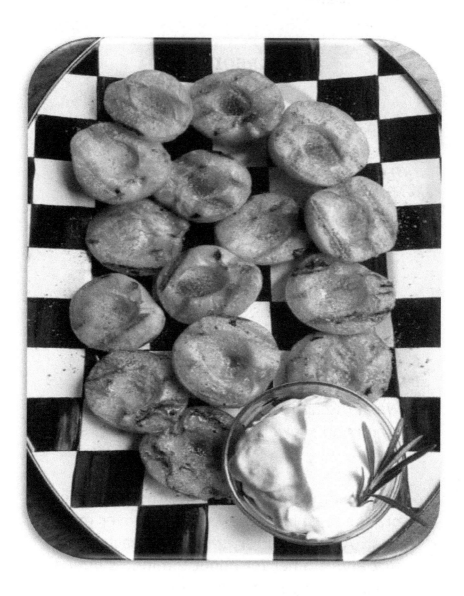

SCHUPFNUDELN WITH POPPY SEEDS AND ORANGE SAUCE

> ➢ **Servings:4**

INGREDIENTS

- ✓ 1 Tbsp Butter
- ✓ 2 Pc Eggs
- ✓ 150 g Flour
- ✓ 500 g floury potatoes
- ✓ 100 g Poppy
- ✓ 7 Pc Oranges
- ✓ 1 prize Salt
- ✓ 1 TL Food starch
- ✓ 60 g Sugar

PREPARATION

- ❖ Boil the potatoes in lightly salted water. Then peel and press through the potato press.

- ❖ Spread on a floured surface, let cool down briefly and then knead with the eggs, flour and a pinch of salt.

❖ Shape the pasta out of the dough and let it rest.

❖ In the meantime, fillet the oranges with a sharp knife and collect the juice. Mix the corn starch with a little orange juice, then bring to the boil with the remaining orange juice and sugar. Finally, briefly add the orange fillets.

❖ Now gradually cook the potato noodles in salted water until they float to the surface and then skim them off. Then rinse in cold water and fry in a little butter.

❖ Spread on plates, drizzle with orange sauce and serve sprinkled with poppy seeds.

VEGETABLE SNACKS

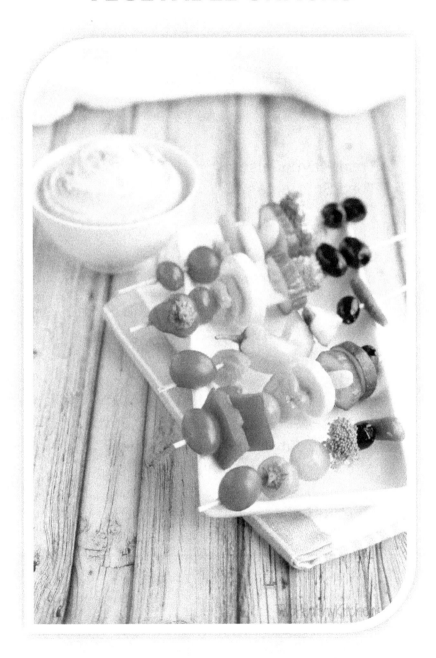

CLASSIC EGG SALAD

INGREDIENTS

- ✓ 8 Pc Eggs
- ✓ 2 Tbsp Mayonnaise
- ✓ 2 Tbsp Sour cream
- ✓ 0.5 TL Mustard
- ✓ 1 Tbsp Vinegar
- ✓ 1 prize Salt
- ✓ 1 prize Pepper from the grinder)

PREPARATION

- ❖ For the classic egg salad, first boil the eggs hard in a saucepan with water for around 10 minutes. Then lift it out of the pot and rinse in cold water, peel and chop into small pieces.

- ❖ Now mix the mayonnaise with salt, pepper, vinegar and sour cream well in a bowl. Mix in the eggs and let them steep in the refrigerator for three hours.

- ❖ After steeping in the refrigerator, season the salad again with salt, pepper and possibly a little mustard.

QUICK BAKED APPLE RINGS

> **Servings:4**

INGREDIENTS

✓ 2 Pc Apples (large, crumbly)

Ingredients for the dough

✓ 250 g Flour
✓ 1 prize Salt
✓ 200 ml Milk
✓ 2 Pc Eggs

Ingredients for frying

✓ 200 ml Oil

PREPARATION

❖ For the quick baked apple rings, first put the flour in a bowl, add salt, milk and egg, stir well so that a thick dough is formed.

❖ Peel the apples, remove the core and cut into rings approx. 1 cm thick. Drizzle lightly with lemon.

❖ Let the fat get hot in a pan. Dip the apple rings in the batter and fry in the hot fat. Turn more often, as soon as they are golden brown, remove from the pan and drain on kitchen paper.

❖ Dust with icing sugar while it is still hot and serve.

VEGETABLE PATTIES

✓ **Servings:4**

INGREDIENTS

- ✓ 1 Pc Zucchini
- ✓ 1 Pc Onions
- ✓ 1 Pc Egg
- ✓ 120 g Flour
- ✓ 1 prize Parsley, chopped
- ✓ 1 prize Pepper
- ✓ 1 prize Salt
- ✓ 100 ml Oil for the pan
- ✓ 3 Pc Potatoes
- ✓ 160 g Celery
- ✓ 2 Pc Carrots
- ✓ 100 g Canned corn

PREPARATION

- ❖ First cook the potatoes in a saucepan with salted water for around 15-20 minutes, then drain, peel and mash with a fork.

- ❖ In the meantime, peel the zucchini, carrots and celery and cut into small cubes.

❖ Then mix the chopped vegetables with the potato mixture.

❖ Now peel the onions, chop them finely and sweat in hot oil until translucent.

❖ Then stir in the roasted onions and corn, as well as egg and flour into the potato mixture and season to taste with salt, pepper and finely chopped parsley.

❖ Using a large spoon, prick a portion out of the mixture and shape it into patties (preferably with wet hands).

❖ Fry the patties in hot oil until golden brown on both sides.

VEGETARIAN CHILI

> **Servings:4**

INGREDIENTS

- ✓ 1 Pc Onion
- ✓ 4 Pc Garlic cloves
- ✓ 2 Pc Paprika (colored)
- ✓ 200 g Kidney beans (can)
- ✓ 150 g Corn (can)
- ✓ 400 g Tomatoes (diced, can)
- ✓ 400 g Lentils (can)
- ✓ 3 Tbsp Tomato paste
- ✓ 3 Tbsp Water
- ✓ 0.5 TL Cayenne pepper
- ✓ 1 TL Salt
- ✓ 1 Tbsp Paprika powder
- ✓ 1 Msp Chili
- ✓ 1 shot Sopy sauce
- ✓ 3 Tbsp Olive oil

PREPARATION

- ❖ For the vegetarian chilli, first peel the onion and garlic. Wash, clean and chop the peppers. Drain the corn, beans and lentils in a colander.

❖ Sauté the garlic, paprika and onion in a saucepan with oil, then stir in the tomato paste and deglaze with a little water. Now stir in the tomatoes, peppers, corn, lentils and beans.

❖ The chilli is now seasoned with salt, cayenne pepper, paprika powder, sopy sauce and chilli powder.

❖ Now let the whole thing simmer for about 20 minutes, stirring frequently.

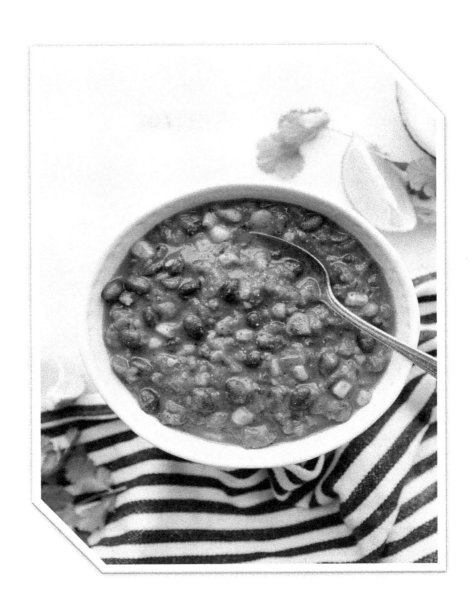

COLE SLAW - AMERICAN COLESLAW

> ➤ **Servings:4**

INGREDIENTS

- ✓ 0.5 kpf White cabbage
- ✓ 250 g Carrots
- ✓ 1 Pc Onion
- ✓ 1 TL Salt
- ✓ 1 prize Pepper
- ✓ Ingredients for the dressing
- ✓ 2 cups Sour cream
- ✓ 2 Tbsp Wine vinegar
- ✓ 1 Tbsp Sugar
- ✓ 1 Tbsp Mayonnaise
- ✓ 1 shot Lemon juice

PREPARATION

❖ First slice the white cabbage finely and mix with salt, let the mixture stand for 1 ½ hours to remove the liquid from the white cabbage.

- ❖ Then squeeze everything out vigorously with the balls of your hands and allow to drain. Grate the carrots, peel and dice the onion and add.
- ❖ For the dressing, mix the sour cream, mayonnaise, wine vinegar, lemon juice and sugar and mix everything well with the vegetables.

- ❖ Season the salad with salt and pepper again and cover and let it steep in the refrigerator for at least 3 hours.

POT DUMPLINGS WITH BREADCRUMBS

> **Servings:4**

INGREDIENTS

- ✓ 1 cups Curd cheese (fine, 250 g)
- ✓ 1 Pc Eggs
- ✓ 1 prize Salt
- ✓ 3 Tbsp Flour
- ✓ 3 Tbsp Semolina
- ✓ 3 Tbsp Butter
- ✓ 3 Tbsp Crumbs
- ✓ 1 Tbsp Sugar

PREPARATION

- ❖ For the pot dumplings with crumbs, first work the curd, egg, flour, semolina and salt into a smooth dough, then leave to rest for 10 minutes.

- ❖ In the meantime, bring a saucepan of salted water to the boil and use two spoons to form dumplings from the dough. Let the dumplings simmer in boiling water for about 15 minutes.

❖ In the meantime, melt the butter in a pan, add the crumbs and sugar and toast. Lift the dumplings out of the water with the slotted spoon and roll them in the butter crumbs.

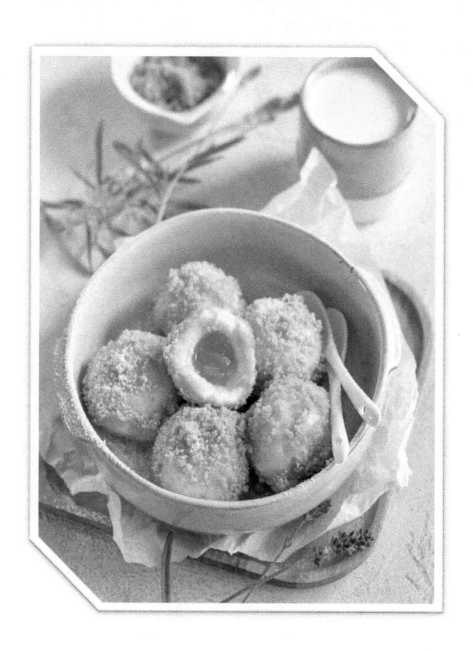

SPINACH LASAGNE WITH BECHAMEL SAUCE

> **Servings:4**

INGREDIENTS

- ✓ 2 Pc Onion
- ✓ 4 Pc Garlic cloves
- ✓ 600 g Spinach - TK
- ✓ 1 Msp Nutmeg
- ✓ 250 g Feta
- ✓ 120 g Cheese (grated)
- ✓ 16 Pc Lasagna sheets
- ✓ 1 Tbsp Oil for the mold
- ✓ 2 Tbsp Oil
- ✓ 1 prize Pepper
- ✓ 1 prize Salt
- ✓ Ingredients for the sauce
- ✓ 50 g Butter
- ✓ 50 g Flour
- ✓ 0.5 l Milk
- ✓ 0.5 l Soup
- ✓ 1 Msp Nutmeg
- ✓ 1 prize Pepper
- ✓ 1 prize Salt

PREPARATION

❖ For the spinach lasagna with bechamel sauce, first preheat the oven to 200 degrees top / bottom heat and coat an ovenproof dish with oil. Finely dice the feta.

❖ Then peel and finely chop the onions and garlic. Sweat both in a little oil in a saucepan. Add the still frozen spinach and thaw. Season with salt, pepper and nutmeg.

❖ For the bechamel sauce, melt the butter in a saucepan, then stir in the flour. Gradually pour in the milk and the soup and stir well so that no lumps form. Season with salt, pepper and nutmeg and simmer for a few minutes.

❖ Now alternately layer the sauce, lasagne sheets, spinach and feta in the baking dish. Start and finish with sauce. Finally sprinkle the cheese over the lasagne and bake in the oven for 35 minutes.

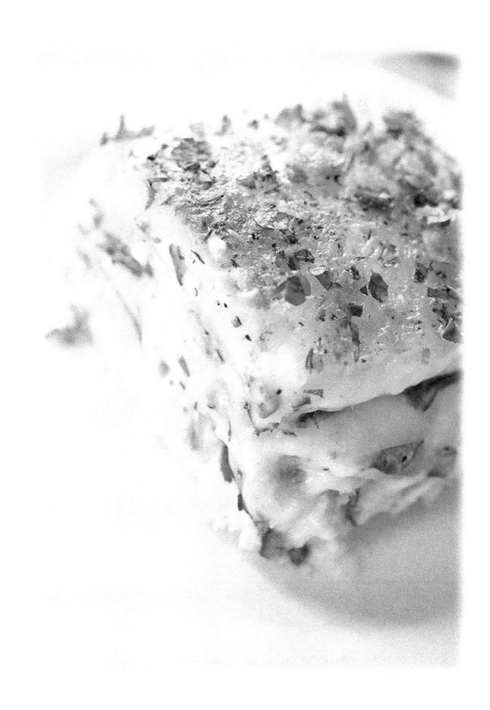

TURKISH FALAFEL

> **Servings:4**

INGREDIENTS

- ✓ 250 g Chickpeas (dried)
- ✓ 1 Federation Corinander
- ✓ 1 Pc Onion
- ✓ 3 Pc Garlic cloves
- ✓ 1 TL Cumin
- ✓ 2 Tbsp Lemon juice
- ✓ 1 prize Pepper from the grinder)
- ✓ 0.5 TL Salt
- ✓ 5 Tbsp Oil (for frying)

PREPARATION

❖ For the Turkish falafel, soak the chickpeas in plenty of water the day before. Drain the water the next day.

❖ Then wash the coriander, drain well and chop finely. Peel and finely dice the garlic and onion.

Puree the uncooked chickpeas with the hand blender. Add coriander, garlic and onion and puree everything finely. Season with salt, pepper and cumin, add the lemon juice and mix everything well.

❖ Heat the oil in a deep pan. Then shape balls out of the mixture and bake the balls until they are golden brown. Drain on paper towels before serving.

CONCLUSION

For a balanced vegetarian lifestyle, it is not enough to omit meat and sausages. Vegetarians should know how to put their food together in such a way that the ingredients are optimally utilized and complement each other.

Variety in the menu protects against an overly one-sided diet.

Without meat, the combination of different proteins is important. Vegetable protein from bread, cereal flakes, vegetables, legumes or potatoes combined with animal protein from milk or eggs is particularly valuable for our body. Experts also speak of a high biological value. Useful combinations include potatoes with eggs or milk, for example as a farmer's breakfast or jacket potatoes with quark, cereals with legumes such as lentil stew with bread or cereals and milk such as muesli.

Even if the fairy tale about iron-containing spinach still holds true, it is correct: iron from meat-containing foods is particularly well absorbed by our body. But even without meat, you can get your necessary iron ration if you make a sensible choice. Whole grain bread, millet, or certain vegetables, such as beetroot or green leafy vegetables, are iron-rich, meatless alternatives. Important: Consuming foods containing vitamin C such as orange juice at the same time improves iron absorption.

The food should be fresh and as wholesome as possible. Processed products often contain less valuable nutrients.

Milk, dairy products and eggs provide our bodies with nutrients that plant-based foods cannot adequately supply.

Pregnant women should supply their bodies with sufficient folic acid. Good sources of this vitamin include kale, spinach, fennel and mung beans.

Vitamin B12 is mainly found in meat. Our body needs it, for example, for blood formation. Alternatively, fortified foods such as soy milk are suitable.

Women with heavy menstrual bleeding should pay particular attention to their iron balance.

The supply of critical nutrients - such as vitamin B12 or vitamin D - should be checked regularly by a doctor.

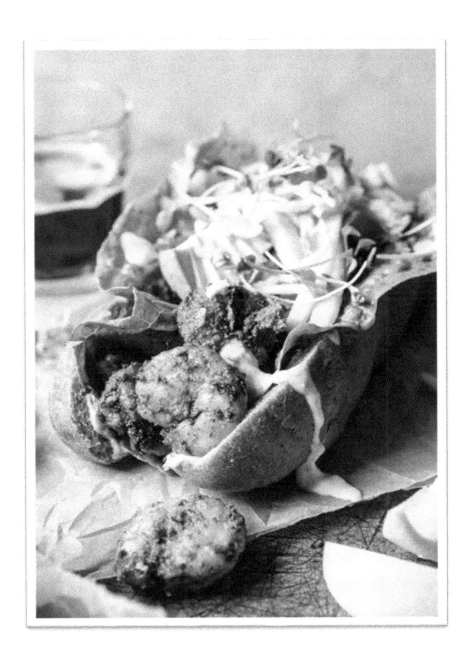